Beef Lc

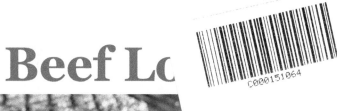

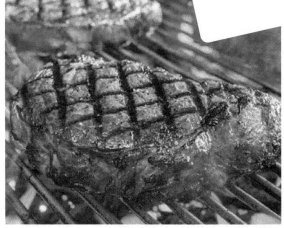

Cookbook

Delice your dinner with these quick and easy recipes for beginners and advanced. Eat your loved red meat, with all the benefits of a detox and healthy lifestyle. Grill and stew. US to Thailand. Try this low-budget and mouth-watering book!

Dorian Gravy

Table of Contents

Welcome, dear hungry buddy!

This is my offer to your cooking style.

This cookbook is the realization of my research on how to eat tasty and healthy food at the meantime.
My purpose is to increase your energies and to let you live a lighter life, without the junk of the globalised kitchen.

In here, you'll find my knowledge on how to create delicious dishes with beef.

Jump into a worldwide discovery of good food and natural-feed animals, with many recipes for a varied diet.

Nevertheless, you'll learn new techniques, discover tastes of all around the world and improve your skills.
Let yourself be inspired by the worldwide traditions, twisted by a proper chef.

Each of these dishes is thought to:

1 – Let you understand how to work with the meat of beef

This majestic animal is presented in various dishes of different cultures, to show you how the same ingredient can change from dish to dish.

2 – Balance your weight with different cooking methods

As soon as you learn different ways to cook your meat, you'll discover an entire world of new ideas.
Beef will never bore you again!

3 – Amaze your friends starting from the smell

Once your friends will come to dinner, they will be in love with your food even before to see your creation.

Beef Recipes

"I love beef steak
And to respect what I eat.
Add some gravyfull ladle,
Am gonna eat it double."

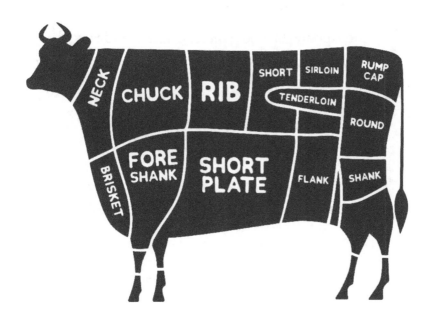

Beef Tartare

Serves 6 pax

Ingredients

- 4 dashes Worcestershire sauce
- 2 dashes hot sauce
- 3/4 teaspoon crushed chile flakes
- 3 teaspoons Dijon mustard
- 2 tablespoons finely chopped red onion
- 2 teaspoons brined capers, drained and rinsed
- 1 medium oil-packed anchovy, rinsed and minced
- 2 large egg yolks
- 10 ounces USDA prime beef tenderloin, cut into small dice, covered, and refrigerated
- 4 teaspoons olive oil
- 2 tablespoons finely chopped Italian parsley leaves

Procedure

1. Combine anchovies (if using), capers, and mustard in a nonreactive bowl.
2. Using a fork or theback of a spoon, mash ingredients until evenly combined; mix in egg yolks.
3. Use a rubber spatula to fold remaining ingredients into mustard mixture until thoroughlycombined. Season well with salt and freshly ground black pepper.
4. Serve immediately with toast points or french fries.

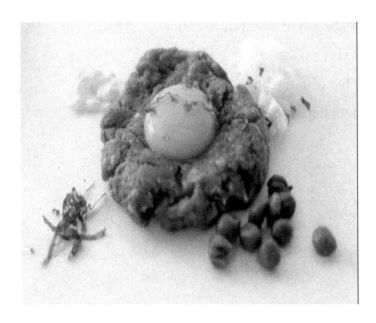

Meat Loaf

Serves 8 pax

Ingredients

- 1 Egg
- 1 tsp Dried oregano
- 1.5 lbs lean ground beef
- 0.5 cup Ground flaxseeds
- 1 Onion
- 3 Tbsp Worcestershire sauce
- 2 cloves Garlic
- 1 tsp Mustard powder
- 0.33 cups Ketchup

Procedure

1. Set the oven temperature at 350° Fahrenheit.

2. Whisk together the ketchup, mustard powder, garlic, and 2 Tbsp. Worcestershire sauce. Place it to the side for now.

3. In another mixing container, combine the remaining 1 Tbsp. Worcestershire sauce with the onion, flaxseeds, ground beef, oregano, egg, and 2 Tbsp. of the ketchup mixture. Press the mixture into the pan coated with nonstick spray.

4. Bake until the center is no longer pink and at least 160°F, about 1 hour. Spread the remaining ketchup mixture over the top of the meatloaf and bake for another 10 minutes.

Roman saltimbocca

Serves 4 pax

Ingredients

- 8 fresh sage leaves, plus extra sage for garnish
- 1 cup all-purpose flour
- 4 thin sliced 5-ounce cutlets of veal
- 2 tablespoons dry white wine
- 1/4 cup chicken broth
- Lemon wedges, for garnish
- 4 slices thin sliced prosciutto
- Salt and freshly ground black pepper
- 2 tablespoons extra-virgin olive oil
- 2 tablespoons unsalted butter

Procedure

1. Place veal cutlets side by side on a sheet of plastic wrap. Place one slice of prosciutto on top of each cutlet Cover with a second sheet of plastic wrap.

2. Gently flatten the cutlets with a rolling pin. Roll until cutlets are 1/4 inch thick and the prosciutto sticks to the veal.

3. Remove the plastic wrap. Place 2 sage leaves atop the center of each cutlet. Thread a toothpick through the veal to keep the prosciutto and sage in place.

4. Put flour in a shallow platter. Season to taste with salt and pepper. Mix with a fork to combine and then dredge the veal in the seasoned flour. Shake off any excess flour.

5. Heat the oil with 1 tablespoon of butter in a large skillet on medium heat. Place the cutlets in the skillet, prosciutto-side down. Cook for 3 minutes until prosciutto is crisp. Turn and sauté for 2 minutes, until golden. Remove cutlets to serving plates. Take out toothpicks and keep plates warmed.

6. Add the wine to the skillet. Stir to bring out the veal flavors from the pan. Heat to reduction for 1 minute. Add chicken broth and remaining tablespoon of butter. Swirl the skillet until butter blends in. Season to taste with salt and pepper.

7. Pour sauce over the saltimbocca. Garnish with remaining sage leaves and lemon wedges.

8. Serve immediately.

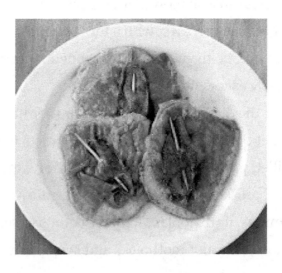

Sriracha Meatballs

Serves 8 pax

- 3 tbsp Coconut nectar
- 2 Eggs
- 3 tbsp Rice vinegar
- 1/2 tsp Sesame oil
- 3 tbsp Soy sauce
- 1/4 cup Sriracha
- 2 Zucchini
- 2 lbs Ground beef
- Salt and pepper to taste
- 4 cups Quinoa
- 1 cup Breadcrumbs
- 2 Carrots
- 3 Garlic cloves
- 1/2 tsp Garlic powder
- 1/4 cup Green onions

Procedure

1. These meatballs cook best at 375° F, so prepare your oven accordingly.

2. Stir the quinoa into eight cups of water. Pour into a pot and get it boiling. Once boiling, reduce heat to allow the quinoa to simmer. Remove from heat once all the water has been absorbed.

3. Take this time to prepare your vegetables according to the ingredient list details. Once done, toss the vegetables into the quinoa pot and stir. Cover and let the vegetables soften. Remove from heat when done.

4. Place a parchment paper blanket on a baking tray, so it is ready to bake. Place the ground beef into a large dish and crack in the eggs and stir in the breadcrumbs. Toss in the green onion, garlic powder, pepper, and salt. Using your hands, knead the ingredients together until fully incorporated.

5. Form 40 meatballs and arrange them on the baking tray, giving them enough space so none touch. Stick the meatballs into the oven and bake for 20 minutes, checking for brownness and doneness.
6. While baking, pour sriracha, coconut nectar, soy sauce, rice vinegar, ginger, sesame oil, and garlic into a small pot. Whisk together until emulsified and place the pot over a moderate heat. Slowly allow the mixture to a boil. Stir regularly.
7. Once boiled, remove the pot from heat. Also, pull the meatballs out of the oven. Coat them with the glaze, making sure to cover them completely in it.
8. Serve the meatballs with a side of quinoa. Garnish with sesame seeds and green onion slices.

Roast Beef Roll-Ups

Serves 6 pax

Ingredients

- 1 tbsp Olive oil - ex.virgin
- 1 tbsp Red wine vinegar
- 6 Romaine lettuce leaves
- Six 10" Whole wheat flour tortillas
- 1 cup Tomato
- 0.25 tsp Fresh ground black pepper
- 1 tsp Cumin
- 1 cup Red bell pepper
- 12 oz. Thin sliced roast beef

Procedure

1. Tear six pieces of foil or waxed paper, each 15". Place a tortilla on each piece.

2. Top each tortilla with a lettuce leaf. Place 2 oz. of roast beef on each piece of lettuce.

3. Dice the peppers and tomatoes.

4. In a small-sized mixing container, mix and toss the tomatoes, red peppers, olive oil, vinegar, pepper, and cumin. Place equal portions of the tomato mixture over the beef.

5. Roll the foil or waxed paper over the tortilla to encase the filling. Roll until the tortilla is completely rolled up with the filling.

6. Fold the excess foil or paper over the bottom and top of each rollup.

7. Peel back the paper or foil to eat.

Thai Beef Sticks

Serves 12 pax

Ingredients

- 1 tsp Black pepper
- 2 cloves Garlic minced
- 12 Bamboo skewers
- 2 Limes, each cut into 6 wedges
- 1 cup Cilantro chopped
- 2 tsp Splenda
- 1 cup Basil
- 2 lbs Lean beef tenderloin, cut into 1" chunks
- 2 stalks Lemongrass
- 2 tbsp Soy sauce

Procedure

1. Soak the dozen wooden skewers in warm water for at least 1/2 hour before using them.

2. Combine the garlic, black pepper, soy sauce, lemongrass, and Splenda, stirring well. Add the beef and cover with a layer of plastic wrap or foil. Pop it into the fridge for one to four hours.

3. Heat the grill. Spear the beef on the 12 skewers, then discard the marinade. Grill the skewers for five minutes per side.

4. Garnish with basil, cilantro, and lime wedges.

5. Serve.

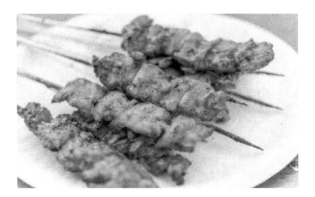

Coffee-Rubbed Steak

Serves 6 pax

Ingredients

- 1 Tbsp. + 0.5 tsp Espresso or instant coffee powder
- 1 Tbsp. + 0.5 tsp Smoked paprika
- 1.25 tsp Chili powder
- 2 Tbsp Olive oil
- 26 oz Lean New York strip steak
- 1 Tbsp. + 0.5 tsp Onion powder
- 0.5 Tbsp Brown sugar

Procedure

1. Combine the brown sugar, chili powder, paprika, onion powder, and espresso powder, then spread mixture on both sides of the steak, pressing it into the meat.

2. Prepare a large nonstick skillet to warm the oil using the medium temperature setting. Cook the steak for five minutes per side, until the inside temperature is 125° Fahrenheit for rare and 145° Fahrenheit for medium-rare, making sure the spices don't burn.

3. Arrange the steak on a cutting board and pour the pan juices over it. Let it sit for 10 minutes, then slice thin.

Chiang Mai Beef

Serves 5 pax

Ingredients

- 1 tablespoon dried small chilies
- 1 tablespoon vegetable oil
- 1 pound lean ground beef
- 1 tablespoon chopped garlic
- 3 cups water
- 3 tablespoons soy sauce
- 3 tablespoons Fish sauce
- 5 cups uncooked long-grained rice
- 2 green onions, trimmed and cut

Procedure

1. In a big deep cooking pan, bring the water to its boiling point, then mix in the rice. Cover, decrease the heat to low, and cook twenty minutes.

2. Place the cooked rice in a big mixing container and let cool completely. Put in the ground beef and soy sauce to the rice, mixing meticulously.

3. Split the rice-beef mixture into 8 to 12 equivalent portions, depending on the size you prefer, and form them into loose balls. Cover each ball in foil, ensuring to secure them well. Steam the rice balls for twenty-five to thirty minutes or until thoroughly cooked.

4. While the rice is steaming, heat the vegetable oil in a small frying pan. Put in the garlic and the dried chilies and sauté until the garlic is golden. Move the garlic and the chilies to a paper towel to drain.

5. To serve, remove the rice packets from the foil, slightly smash them, and put on serving plates. Pass the garlic-chili mixture, the green onions, and the fish sauce separately to be used as condiments at the table.

Veal Cordon Bleu

Serves 5 pax

Ingredients

- 6 slices smoked ham, 1/8-inch-thick
- 1 cup white breadcrumbs
- 3 teaspoons salt
- 3 tablespoons extra virgin olive oil
- 1 lemon cut into 6 wedges
- 6 sprigs fresh parsley
- 12 - 2 ounces veal cutlets, 1/8" thick
- 12 ounces Emmenthal cheese
- 1 teaspoon fresh ground black pepper
- 1 cup all-purpose flour
- 3 large eggs
- 3 tablespoons unsalted butter

Procedure

1. If cutlets are too thick, pound them down to 1/8". Place between two sheets of plastic wrap and use flat side of meat pounder until 1/8" thick. Shave cheese thin enough for a double layer for 6 cutlets.

2. Pat 2 equal cutlets dry on a clean work surface. Place 1 slice of ham on cutlet. Trim ham to 1/4" smaller than veal. Place 2 layers of cheese on ham. Top with second cutlet. Lightly pound the 1/4" border at cutlet edges until sealed. Repeat for 5 more veal sandwiches.

3. Line baking sheet with wax paper. Mix breadcrumbs, 1 teaspoon salt, and 1/2 teaspoon pepper in baking dish. Stir together flour, 1 teaspoon salt, and 1/2 teaspoon pepper in second baking dish.

4. Whisk eggs with remaining salt and pepper in third baking dish. Dredge 1 veal sandwich in flour. Brush off excess flour. Dip in egg to coat. When excess egg drips off, dredge in breadcrumbs and pat until coating sticks.

5. Place coated veal on a rack set on a baking sheet. Repeat dredge and coating for remaining veal sandwiches. Chill 1 hour, uncovered. Let stand 30 minutes at room temperature prior to cooking.

6. Heat 1 tablespoon butter and 1 tablespoon olive oil in heavy skillet on medium-high heat. When foaming stops, add 2 veal sandwiches. Lower heat to medium. Cook, 4 minutes, turning once. Cutlet is done when golden both sides.

7. Transfer veal to serving plates. Wipe skillet clean. Repeat process twice to cook 4 more veal sandwiches in remaining butter and olive oil.

Loubia

Serves 6 pax

Ingredients

- 1 (12- to 16-ounce) lamb shank
- 1 onion, chopped
- 1 pound dried great Northern beans
- 1/4 teaspoon cayenne pepper
- 1/2 cup dry white wine
- 1 red bell pepper, stemmed, seeded, and chopped
- 1 tablespoon extra-virgin olive oil
- 6 tablespoons tomato paste
- 2 teaspoons ground cumin
- 2 teaspoons paprika
- 2 garlic cloves, minced
- 3 cups chicken broth
- 1 teaspoon ground ginger
- 3 tablespoons minced fresh parsley
- Salt and pepper

Procedure

1. Dissolve 3 tablespoons salt in 4 quarts cold water in large container. Put in beans and soak at room temperature for minimum 8 hours or for maximum 24 hours. Drain and wash thoroughly.

2. Place oven rack to lower-middle position and pre-heat your oven to 350 degrees. Pat lamb dry using paper towels and sprinkle with salt and pepper. Heat oil in a

3. Dutch oven on moderate to high heat until just smoking. Brown lamb on all sides, 10 to fifteen minutes; move to plate. Pour off all but 2 tablespoons fat from pot.

4. Put in onion and bell pepper to fat left in pot and cook on moderate heat till they become tender and lightly browned, 5 to 7 minutes. Mix in tomato paste, garlic, paprika, cumin, ginger, cayenne, and 1/8 teaspoon pepper and cook until aromatic, approximately half a minute. Mix in wine, scraping up any browned bits. Mix in broth, 1 cup water, and beans and bring to boil.

5. Nestle lamb into beans along with any accumulated juices. Cover, move pot to oven, and cook until fork slips easily in and out of lamb and beans are tender, 11/2 to 13/4 hours, stirring every 30 minutes.

6. Move lamb to slicing board, allow to cool slightly, then shred into bite-size pieces using 2 forks; discard excess fat and bone. Stir shredded lamb and parsley into beans and sprinkle with salt and pepper to taste. Adjust consistency with extra hot water as required.

7. Serve, drizzling individual portions with extra oil.

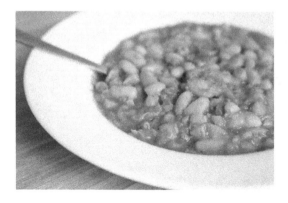

Creamed Horseradish

Serves 6 pax

Ingredients

- 1 tablespoon Champagne vinegar
- 1 tablespoon chives, minced
- 1 teaspoon salt
- 1 teaspoon fresh ground black pepper
- 1/4 teaspoon red chile powder
- 2 cups crème fraîche
- 1/2 cup fresh horseradish, peeled and grated
- 1 tablespoon scallions, minced

Procedure

1. Mix all ingredients well in a bowl.
2. Serve cold.

Lamb Filled Zucchini

Serves 5 pax

Ingredients

- 2/3 cup chicken broth
- 1 onion, chopped fine
- 1/4 cup dried apricots, chopped fine
- 1/2 cup medium-grind bulgur, rinsed
- 2 tablespoons minced fresh parsley
- 4 zucchini (8 ounces each), halved along the length and seeded
- 8 ounces ground lamb
- Salt and pepper
- 2 tablespoons pine nuts, toasted
- 2 tablespoons plus 1 teaspoon extra-virgin olive oil
- 2 teaspoons ras el hanout
- 4 garlic cloves, minced

Procedure

1. Adjust oven racks to upper-middle and lowest positions, place rimmed baking sheet on lower rack, and pre-heat your oven to 400 degrees.

2. Brush cut sides of zucchini with 2 tablespoons oil and sprinkle with salt and pepper. Lay zucchini cut side down in hot sheet and roast until slightly softened and skins are wrinkled, eight to ten minutes. Remove zucchini from oven and flip cut side up on sheet; set aside.

3. In the meantime, heat remaining 1 teaspoon oil in a big saucepan on moderate to high heat until just smoking.

4. Put in lamb, 1/2 teaspoon salt, and 1/4 teaspoon pepper and cook, breaking up meat with wooden spoon, until browned, 3 to 5 minutes. Use a slotted spoon to move lamb to paper towel–lined plate.

5. Pour off all but 1 tablespoon fat from saucepan. Put in onion to fat left in saucepan and cook on moderate heat till they become tender, approximately five minutes.

6. Mix in garlic and ras el hanout and cook until aromatic, approximately half a minute. Mix in broth, bulgur, and apricots and bring to simmer. Decrease heat to low, cover, and simmer gently until bulgur is tender, 16 to 18 minutes.

7. Remove from the heat, lay clean dish towel underneath lid and let pilaf sit for about ten minutes.

8. Put in pine nuts and parsley to pilaf and gently fluff with fork to combine. Sprinkle with salt and pepper to taste.

9. Pack each zucchini half with bulgur mixture, about 1/2 cup per zucchini half, mounding excess.

10. Place baking sheet on upper rack and bake zucchini until heated through, about 6 minutes.

11. Serve.

Oxtail Soup

Serves 6 pax

Ingredients

- 2 tablespoons beef drippings
- 2 yellow onions, minced
- 2 pounds oxtails
- 1/2 cup plus 2 tablespoons flour
- 1 stalk celery, diced
- 1/3 cup port wine
- 2 quarts water
- 2 tablespoons tomato paste
- 1/2 teaspoon thyme
- 3 cloves
- 2 sprigs parsley
- 2 teaspoons salt
- 1/4 teaspoon fresh ground black pepper
- 1 bay leaf
- 2 carrots, diced

Procedure

1. Cut oxtails into 1" segments. Trim fat. Dredge oxtail segments in 1/2 cup flour.

2. Cook in beef drippings in large pot on high heat. When browned, set aside oxtails on paper towels to drain.

3. Reduce heat to medium. Add onions and sauté 10 minutes. When onions are golden, sprinkle in remaining 2 tablespoons flour and mix well. Cook until lightly browned.

4. Slowly add water and stir in tomato paste, salt, and pepper. Tie bay leaf, thyme, cloves, and parsley into a cheesecloth sachet. Add to pot.

5. Return previously set aside oxtails to pot. Simmer covered 3 hours. Oxtails are done when meat is fork tender. Let cool, skim fat and remove herb sachet.

6. Separate oxtail meat from bones. Cut meat into bite-size pieces. Return meat to pot. Add carrots and celery. Simmer covered 15 minutes. When carrots are tender, add port wine.

7. Once emulsified, serve.

Crisp Pastry

Serves 6 pax

Ingredients

- 6 tablespoons water
- 20 ounces puff pastry
- 1 pinch of salt
- 6 egg yolks
- 2 tablespoons light cream

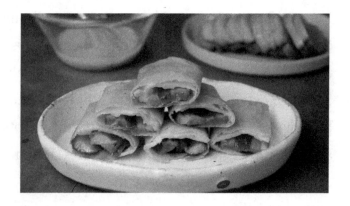

Procedure

1. Roll puff pastry dough out to 1/8" thickness. Cut 6 rounds of pastry a little bigger than the cooking ramekins.
2. Fill ramekins until 3/4 full of oxtail soup (recipe above). Mix 2 egg yolks and 2 tablespoons water into a wash. Rub ramekin rims with egg wash.
3. Cover ramekins with dough rounds. Pull slightly on edges. Do not let dough touch the soup. Refrigerate 1 hour. Remove ramekins from refrigerator 15 minutes before baking. Preheat oven to 400°F.
4. Whisk remaining 4 egg yolks, water, light cream and salt together in a small bowl. Egg wash is blended when thick enough to apply without drips. Brush pastry with egg wash.
5. Bake 20 minutes. Oxtail en croute is done when pastry is golden-brown.
6. Serve hot.

Beef Medallions & Mushroom Sauce

Serves 12 pax

Ingredients

- 4 garlic cloves, chopped
- 2/3 cup shallots, chopped
- 1 pound beef tenderloin
- 1 cup sliced mushrooms
- Salt and fresh ground black pepper
- 4 tablespoons butter
- 1 teaspoon dried thyme
- 1 tablespoon all-purpose flour
- 3 cups beef broth
- 2 cups dry red wine

Procedure

1. Cut tenderloin crosswise into 12 equal rounds. Pound beef rounds until they form flat 1/4 -inch thick medallions. Season lightly with salt and pepper.

2. Melt 2 tablespoons butter in large skillet on medium-high heat. Sauté medallions 2 minutes until browned. Turn medallions over and sauté 2 more minutes to brown other side. Set aside medallions.

3. Melt 2 tablespoons butter in same skillet. Add mushrooms, garlic, shallots and thyme. Sauté 3 minutes until tender. Add flour. Stir 1 minute. Add broth and wine. Boil 12 minutes, stirring occasionally, until sauce thickens and reduces to 11/4 cups.

4. Return medallions to skillet. Heat 1 minute until medallions are hot throughout.

5. Spoon sauce equally over medallions and serve.

Petite Marmite

Serves 6 pax

Ingredients

- 6 whole black peppercorns
- 1/2 teaspoon nutmeg
- Salt and fresh ground black pepper
- teaspoons fresh parsley, chopped
- 4 ounces bone marrow, sliced
- 2 quarts water
- 2 teaspoons chervil
- 1 bay leaf
- 2 cloves garlic, crushed
- 3/4 ounce white cabbage
- 1 cup dry red wine
- 3/4 pound beef, shoulder palette
- 1 pounds chicken breast
- 1 ounce leeks
- 1 ounce carrots
- 3/4 ounce celery root

Procedure

1. Blanch meats 5 to 10 minutes in boiling water. Put beef in stock pot. Cover with water. Simmer 1 hour.
2. Add chicken, peppercorns, bay leaf, garlic and salt. Simmer 40 minutes.
3. Cut vegetables into long thin strips (Julienne). Add vegetables to stock pot and simmer 20 minutes.
4. Remove meats from pot. Cut meats into long thin strips (Julienne). Return meats to stockpot.
5. Bring soup to boil. Add 1 cup dry red wine, bone marrow, parsley, nutmeg and chervil. Season to taste with salt and pepper.

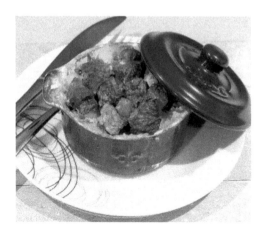

Juicy Rib

Serves 6 pax

Ingredients

- Fresh ground black pepper
- 2 cups dry red wine
- 2 teaspoons fresh rosemary, chopped
- 5 lb bone-in prime rib
- 6 cloves garlic, cut into thin slivers salt
- 4 cups beef stock
- 1 tablespoon fresh thyme, chopped

Procedure

1. Preheat oven to 450°F.
2. Cut shallow slits all over prime rib with tip of sharp knife. Fill each slit with a sliver of garlic. Season generously salt and pepper.
3. Place roast, bones down on roasting rack set inside roasting pan. Insert meat thermometer in center of roast. Avoid fat or bone. Oven sear 10 minutes in 450°F oven.
4. Reduce heat to 350°F. Roast 2 hours until thermometer reads 140°F for medium-rare. (Roast 21/2 hours until thermometer reads 155°F for medium). Remove roast from oven and transfer to cutting board. Cover with foil to keep warm.
5. Place roasting pan of drippings over 2 burners on high heat. Add wine. Cook to a reduction on high heat, stirring pan bottom with wooden spoon.
6. Add beef stock. Cook until au ju reduces in half.
7. Whisk in thyme and rosemary. Season to taste with salt and pepper.
8. Carve roast into thin slices. Serve beef with au jus sauce.

Beef Stuffed Peppers

Serves 4 pax

Ingredients

- 1/2 cup long-grain white rice
- 1/2 teaspoon red pepper flakes
- 3/4 teaspoon ground cardamom
- 1/4 cup currants
- 1/4 cup slivered almonds, toasted and chopped
- 2 teaspoons grated fresh ginger
- 2 teaspoons ground cumin
- 2 garlic cloves, minced
- 2 bell peppers, 1/2 inch trimmed off tops
- 1/4 teaspoon ground cinnamon
- 1 (14.5-ounce) can diced tomatoes
- 1 onion, chopped fine
- 1 tablespoon extra-virgin olive oil
- 10 ounces 90 percent lean ground beef
- 2 ounces feta cheese, crumbled
- 2 teaspoons chopped fresh oregano

Procedure

1. Bring 4 quarts water to boil in large pot. Put in bell peppers and 1 tablespoon salt and cook until just starting to soften, 3 to 5 minutes.
2. Using tongs, remove peppers from pot, drain excess water, and place peppers cut side up on paper towels.
3. Return water to boil, put in rice, and cook until tender, about 13 minutes. Drain rice and move to big container; set aside.
4. Place the oven rack in the centre of the oven and pre-heat your oven to 350 degrees. Heat oil in 12-inch frying pan on moderate to high heat until it starts to shimmer.
5. Put in onion and 1/4 teaspoon salt and cook till they become tender and lightly browned, 5 to 7 minutes.
6. Mix in garlic, ginger, cumin, cardamom, pepper flakes, and cinnamon and cook until aromatic, approximately half a minute.

7. Put in ground beef and cook, breaking up meat with wooden spoon, until no longer pink, about 4 minutes. Remove from the heat, mix in tomatoes and reserved juice, currants, and oregano, scraping up any browned bits.

8. Move mixture to a container with rice. Put in 1/4 cup feta and almonds and gently toss to combine. Sprinkle with salt and pepper to taste.

9. Place peppers cut side up in 8-inch square baking dish. Pack each pepper with rice mixture, mounding filling on top.

10. Bake until filling is heated through, approximately half an hour. Sprinkle remaining 1/4 cup feta over peppers and drizzle with extra oil.

11. Serve.

Lamb Navarin

Serves 6 pax

Ingredients

- 3 cups Campbell's Real Stock Chicken
- 3 garlic cloves, crushed
- 6 fresh thyme sprigs
- 2 tablespoons olive oil
- 2 tablespoons tomato paste
- 1 cup frozen green peas
- 300g green beans, topped
- Crusty bread, to serve
- 1 cup dry white wine
- 2 x 1kg boned rolled lamb shoulders, cut into 4cm
- 2 tablespoons plain flour
- 16 chat potatoes, halved 3 dried bay leaves
- 2 bunches spring onions, ends trimmed
- 2 bunches baby carrots, ends trimmed, peeled

Procedure

1. Heat the oil in a large stockpot over medium-high heat. Add a third of the lamb and cook, turning, for 3-4 minutes or until brown.

2. Transfer to a plate. Repeat, in 2 more batches, with the remaining lamb, reheating the pan between batches.

3. Add the flour, tomato paste and garlic and cook, stirring, for 2 minutes. Remove from heat and whisk in the stock and wine. Add the thyme and bay leaves and bring to the boil over high heat.

4. Return lamb to pan. Reduce heat to low and simmer, covered, stirring occasionally, for 1 hour 10 minutes.

5. Add the potato to the lamb mixture and cook, covered, for 30 minutes. Uncover and cook, stirring occasionally, for 10 minutes or until sauce thickens.

6. Meanwhile, cook the carrots in a large saucepan of boiling water for 3-4 minutes or until tender.

7. Transfer to a plate. Repeat with the spring onions and the beans.
8. Add the carrots, onions, beans and peas to the lamb mixture and cook for 2-3 minutes, or until heated through. Taste and season with salt and pepper.
9. Place the lamb mixture in a large serving dish and serve immediately with crusty bread if desired.

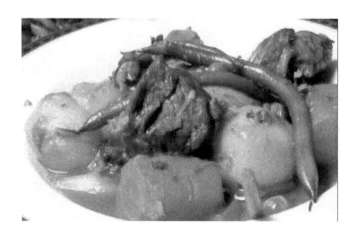

Cambogee Beef

Serves 6 pax

Ingredients

- 2 cups bean sprouts
- 2 moderate-sized russet potatoes, peeled and sliced
- 1/2 cup chopped peanuts
- 1 pound sirloin, trimmed, and slice into bites
- 5 cups Red Curry Cambogee

Procedure

1. In a big deep cooking pan, bring the curry sauce to a simmer.
2. Put in the meat and potatoes and simmer until done to your preference.
3. Decorate using the peanuts and bean sprouts.
4. Serve.

Oxtail Stew

Ingredients

- 1 small cinnamon stick
- 1 tablespoon vegetable oil
- 1 tablespoon whole black peppercorns
- 2 garlic cloves, peeled and crushed
- 1/4 cup chopped cilantro
- 1/2 pound bean sprouts
- 1 (7-ounce) package rice sticks, soaked in hot water
- 1 green onion, trimmed and thinly cut
- 2 limes, cut into wedges
- 2 serrano chilies, seeded and thinly cut
- 2 pounds meaty oxtails
- Freshly ground black pepper to taste
- 2 medium carrots, peeled and julienned
- 2 medium onions
- 2 tablespoons fish sauce
- (1/2-inch) pieces ginger, peeled

Procedure

1. Cut 1 of the onions into 1/4-inch slices. Heat the vegetable oil in a moderate-sized sauté pan on moderate to high heat. Put in the onion slices and sauté until they barely start to brown. Drain the oil from the browned onion and save for later.

2. Slice the rest of the onion into paper-thin slices. Cover using plastic wrap and save for later.

3. Wash the oxtails in cold water and put them in a stock pot. Cover the tails with cold water and bring to its boiling point.

4. Lower the heat and skim any residue that has come to the surface. Let simmer for fifteen minutes.

5. Put in the browned onions, ginger, carrots, cinnamon, star anise, peppercorns, and garlic. Return the stock to a simmer and cook for 6 to 8 hours, putting in water if required. When the broth is done, skim off any additional residue.

6. Take away the oxtails from the pot and allow to cool until easy to handle. Take away the meat from the bones.

7. Position the meat on a platter and decorate it with the cut green onions. Discard the bones.

8. Strain the broth and return to the stove. Put in the fish sauce and black pepper to taste. Keep warm.

9. On a second platter, position the bean sprouts, chopped cilantro, cut chilies, and lime wedges.

10. Bring a pot of water to its boiling point. Plunge the softened rice noodles in the water to heat. Drain.

11. To serve, place a portion of the noodles in each container.

12. Set a tureen of the broth on the table together with the platter of oxtail meat and the platter of accompaniments.

Grilled Beef Tenderloin

Serves 4 pax

Ingredients

- 1 teaspoon fresh garlic, finely chopped
- 1/2 teaspoon fresh ground black pepper
- 4 beef tenderloin steaks
- 1 tablespoon butter
- 1/2 teaspoon chili powder

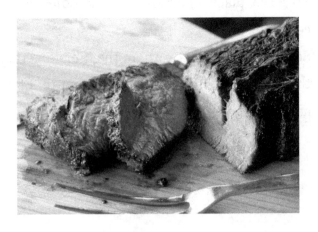

Procedure

1. Place a steak on a cutting board. With a long sharp knife cut the steak horizontally at its mid-point to within a half inch of the other side.

2. Open the two flaps of meat without letting the pieces fall apart. If done correctly steaks resemble butterfly wings. Place the butterflied steak between two sheets of plastic wrap.

3. Beat with a meat mallet to an even thickness. Repeat until all steaks are butterflied.

4. Heat a charcoal grill until coals are ash white.

5. Mix butter, garlic, pepper and chili powder in small bowl. Brush steaks with butter mixture and place on grill.

6. Grill 15 minutes, turning once and brushing intermittently with butter mixture.

7. Let rest 4 minutes and serve.

Honey Baby Carrots

Serves 4 pax

Ingredients

- 3 tablespoons butter
- 2 tablespoons honey
- 2 teaspoons fresh squeezed lemon juice
- 1 pound baby carrots
- 3/4 teaspoon salt
- 1 tablespoon brown sugar
- 1 tsp fresh parsley, chopped for garnish

Procedure

1. Put carrots in a medium saucepan and cover with water. Add salt and bring to boil.

2. Lower heat and cover. Cook 15 minutes on medium-low heat. Carrots are done when tender. Drain and set aside.

3. Melt butter in sautèe pan on medium-low heat. Add honey and brown sugar. Stir until sugar is fully dissolved.

4. Mix in lemon juice and gently stir in carrots. Stir carrots gently until well coated.

5. Continue heating and stirring until carrots are hot and glazed.

6. Garnish with chopped parsley.

7. Serve hot.

Red Potatoes

Ingredients

- 1 head garlic
- 1/4 cup extra virgin olive oil
- Salt and fresh ground black pepper
- 1 pound new red bliss potatoes
- 2 tablespoons chopped parsley
- 1/4 cup water
- 1/4 cup fresh grated parmesan cheese

Procedure

1. Preheat oven to 400°F. Scrub potatoes and cut into halves. Peel garlic and break into cloves.
2. Combine potatoes, olive oil, garlic, salt and pepper in a large bowl. Toss until well coated.
3. Arrange potatoes in a single layer inside roasting pan. Sprinkle with water. Roast 45 minutes. Potatoes are done when tender and golden brown.
4. Toss potatoes and garlic in a serving bowl with cheese and parsley.
5. Serve hot.

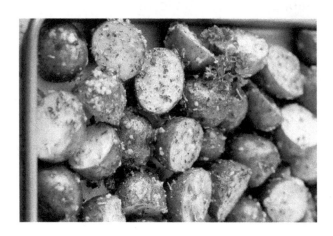

Beef and Lime Sauce

Serves 4 pax

Ingredients

- 1 pound sirloin, trimmed and slice into bites
- 1 tablespoon sugar
- 2 teaspoons freshly ground black pepper, divided
- 5 cloves garlic, crushed
- 1 teaspoon water
- 2 tablespoons lime juice
- 2 tablespoons soy sauce
- 2 tablespoons vegetable oil

Procedure

1. In a container big enough to hold the beef, mix the sugar, 1 teaspoon of black pepper, soy sauce, and garlic.
2. Put in the beef and toss to coat. Cover and let marinate for half an hour
3. In a small serving dish, mix the rest of the black pepper, the lime juice, and the water; set aside.
4. In a big sauté pan, heat the vegetable oil on moderate to high heat. Put in the beef cubes and sauté for about four minutes for medium-rare.
5. This dish may be served either as an appetizer or a main dish:

For the appetizer

1. Mound the beef on a plate lined with lettuce leaves with the lime sauce on the side.
2. Use toothpicks or small forks to immerse the beef into the lime sauce.

For a main dish

1. Toss the beef with the lime sauce to taste.
2. Serve with Jasmine rice.

Freestyle Potatoes

Ingredients

- 1 pound potatoes
- 1 clove garlic, crushed
- 1 large egg, beaten
- 1/4 cup melted butter
- 1 pinch dried dill
- 2 tablespoons heavy cream
- 1/4 teaspoon paprika
- 1 sprig fresh parsley
- 3/4 teaspoon salt
- 1/4 teaspoon fresh ground black pepper
- 1 tablespoon grated Parmesan cheese

Procedure

1. Peel potatoes and cut into cubes. Place cubes in a large stock pot of water.
2. Bring to a boil on medium-high heat. Boil until tender. Drain and return potatoes to stock pot.
3. Whip with an electric mixer. Slowly mix in beaten egg, half of the butter, garlic, dill, grated cheese, heavy cream, salt and pepper.
4. Continue whipping until the smooth. Test consistency and add more milk if needed. Season to taste with salt and pepper.
5. Place whipped potatoes in a pastry bag fitted with a large star tip.
6. Grease a large, greased baking sheet and pipe whipped potatoes into 12 mounds.
7. Drizzle the rest of the butter over the potatoes. Using a pastry brush, dab a little paprika paste lightly onto each potato mound.
8. Garnish with a sprinkling of dried parsley. Preheat oven to 400°F. Bake 20 minutes. Potatoes are done when golden brown at the edges.
9. Remove from oven and serve piping hot.

Roasted Rack of Lamb

Serves 6 pax

Ingredients

- 4 teaspoons fresh chopped rosemary
- 4 cloves garlic, minced salt
- 4 tablespoons extra virgin olive oil
- 2 racks of lamb, Frenched (2 pounds each)
- 2 teaspoons fresh ground black pepper
- 2 teaspoons fresh chopped thyme

Procedure

1. Combine rosemary, thyme, and garlic to make a rubbing mixture. Rub rib racks entirely with herb mixture. Sprinkle with pepper.
2. Place rib racks in a heavy plastic bag. Add olive oil and toss until lamb racks are thoroughly coated. Squeeze air from bag and seal.
3. Refrigerate overnight to marinate. Remove lamb racks from refrigerator 2 hours before cooking to let reach room temperature.
4. Preheat oven to 400°F. Make sharp shallow cuts through the fat at 1" intervals. Sprinkle all over with salt and pepper.
5. Place lamb racks bone side down in roasting pan. Wrap exposed ribs in tin foil. Place pan on center oven rack.
6. Roast 7 minutes at 400°F.
7. Reduce heat to 300°F.
8. Roast 12 minutes at 300°F.

9. Meat is done to President Reagan's preference for rosé when a meat thermometer reads 125°F in the thickest part of the meat. If your preference is for medium rare it should read 135°F.
10. Remove from oven and cover with tin foil. Let stand 10 minutes.
11. Slice between ribs to cut into 2 or 3 lamb chops per guest.
12. Drizzle with California Rosé Wine-Shallots Sauce (recipe follows)
13. Serve with Princess Potatoes and Fennel Gratinée (recipes follow)

Wow Mushrooms

Serves 4 pax

Ingredients

- 1/3 cup sherry
- 1 tablespoon olive oil
- 8 ounces Crimini mushrooms
- 1 tablespoon Worcestershire sauce
- 2 teaspoons fresh thyme

Procedure

1. Heat olive oil in large skillet on medium-high heat. Sauté mushrooms 4 minutes. Stir frequently.
2. Stir in wine, Worcestershire sauce, and thyme. Simmer 3 minutes uncovered.
3. Spoon over steaks

Rosé Wine and Shallots Reduction

Serves 6 pax

Ingredients

- 1 ounce butter
- 1 cup sliced shallots
- 2 tablespoons minced garlic
- 1 bay leaf
- 1 cup California Rosé Wine
- 2 cups veal stock
- 1 ounce butter

Procedure

1. Heat 1/2 ounce butter in a medium saucepan on medium-low heat.
2. Add shallots and garlic. Sauté 5 minutes. Shallots and garlic are done when tender.
3. Add wine and bay leaf. Bring to a boil. Cook until reduced in half.
4. Add veal stock. Cook 20 minutes. Sauce in ready when reduced by 1 cup. Remove from heat and discard bay leaf.
5. Whisk in remaining ounce of butter. Drizzle over Roast Rack of Lamb (recipe above).

Gratined Fennel

Serves 6 pax

Ingredients

- 2 tablespoons unsalted butter salt
- 1 tablespoon fresh ground black pepper
- 3 tablespoons butter
- 1 large shallot, minced
- 3/4 cup red wine
- 3/4 cup breadcrumbs
- 1 cup Pecorino Romano cheese
- 3 tablespoons fresh parsley, chopped
- 3 large garlic cloves, minced
- 5 fresh fennel bulbs, trimmed, cored and sliced
- 1/2 cup low-sodium chicken broth
- 1 teaspoon lemon zest
- 5 tablespoons olive oil
- 1 onion, halved and sliced 1/4" thick
- 1 tablespoon chopped fresh thyme
- 1 teaspoon sea salt

Procedure

1. Lightly oil a baking dish. Heat olive oil in large skillet on medium heat. Sauté onion and garlic 5 minutes. Onion and garlic are done when soft but not browned.
2. Add fennel and heat on medium-high heat. Sauté fennel 15-20 minutes. Stir frequently. Fennel is done when softened and starts to brown.
3. Stir in broth, 2 tablespoons parsley, thyme, sea salt and 1/2 teaspoon pepper. Lower heat to medium-low and simmer 5 minutes. After most of the broth absorbs transfer to baking dish.
4. Preheat oven to 425 F. Let stand at room temperature 1 hour before baking.
5. Melt butter in large skillet on medium heat. Add breadcrumbs and sauté 3 minutes. Breadcrumbs are done when golden brown. Remove from heat and let cool.
6. Stir cheese, 1 tablespoon parsley, and lemon zest into breadcrumbs.

7. Sprinkle breadcrumbs mix over fennel. Bake 20 minutes.

8. Dish is done when gratin is warmed through and topping is toasted golden brown.

9. Serve warm.

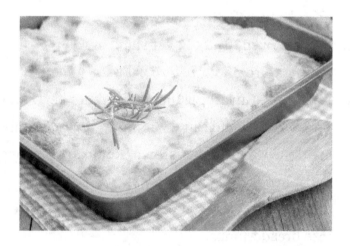

Curry, Beef and Potatoes

Serves 4 pax

Ingredients

- 1/2 cup unsalted roasted peanuts, chopped
- 1/2 cup prepared Massaman Curry Paste
- 1/4 cup Tamarind Concentrate
- 1/2 cup brown sugar
- 1 big onion, chopped
- 1 big russet potato, peeled and slice into bites
- 2 tablespoons vegetable oil
- 7 tablespoons fish sauce
- 4 cups Jasmine rice, cooked in accordance with package direction
- 1 cup chopped fresh pineapple
- 1 pound beef stew meat, cut into bite-sized cubes
- 2 (14-ounce) cans coconut milk

Procedure

1. Heat the oil in a big soup pot on moderate to high heat. Once the oil is hot, brown the meat on all sides. Put in the onion and cook until translucent, approximately two to three minutes.

2. Put in enough water to just cover the meat and onions. Bring to its boiling point, reduce heat, cover, and simmer for thirty to 60 minutes.

3. Put in the potatoes and carry on simmering for fifteen more minutes. (The potatoes will not be fairly thoroughly cooked now.) Strain the solids from the broth, saving for later both.

4. In another soup pot, mix the coconut milk with the curry paste until well mixed. Bring the contents to a simmer on moderate to high heat and cook for two to three minutes.

5. Put in the reserved meat and potato mixture, the sugar, fish sauce, and tamarind, stirring until the sugar dissolves. Put in some of the reserved broth to thin the sauce to desired consistency.

6. Mix in the pineapple and carry on simmering until the potatoes are thoroughly cooked.

7. To serve, place some Jasmine rice in the center of individual serving plates and spoon the stew over the top. Decorate using the chopped peanuts.

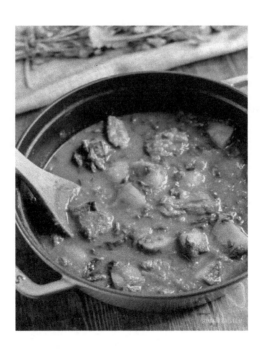

Red Curry Beef

Ingredients

- 1 pound lean beef, cut into fine strips
- 1 tablespoon vegetable oil
- 1/4 cup chopped basil
- 1/2 cup plus 2 tablespoons coconut milk
- 2 tablespoons Red Curry Paste
- 4 cups rice, cooked in accordance with package directions
- Sugar to taste
- 1 green or red sweet pepper, seeded and cubed
- 1 tablespoons fish sauce
- 2 tablespoons roughly ground peanuts

Procedure

1. Heat the oil in a big sauté pan using low heat. Put in the curry paste and cook, stirring continuously, until aromatic, approximately one minute.
2. Mix in the 1/2 cup of coconut milk and bring the mixture to a simmer. Put in the beef strips and poach for five minutes.
3. Put in the peanuts and continue to poach for another five minutes. Put in the fish sauce and sugar to taste. Carry on cooking until the mixture is almost dry, then put in the sweet pepper and basil and cook for 5 more minutes.
4. Serve with rice.

Spicy Sour Beef

Serves 2 pax

Ingredients

- 1 tablespoon lime juice
- 1 teaspoon chopped cilantro
- 1 green onion, trimmed and thinly cut
- 1 tablespoon dark, sweet soy sauce
- 3 tablespoons chopped onion
- Salt and pepper to taste
- 1 tablespoon fish sauce
- 1 teaspoon dried chili powder
- 1 teaspoon honey
- 1 pound sirloin steak

Procedure

1. Make the sauce by meticulously combining the first 8 ingredients. Set aside.
2. Flavor the steak with salt and pepper, then grill or broil it to your preferred doneness.
3. Take away the steak from the grill, cover using foil, and allow to rest for five to ten minutes.
4. Thinly slice the steak, cutting across the grain.
5. Position the pieces on a serving platter or on 1 or 2 dinner plates. Ladle the sauce over the top.
6. Serve with rice and a side vegetable.

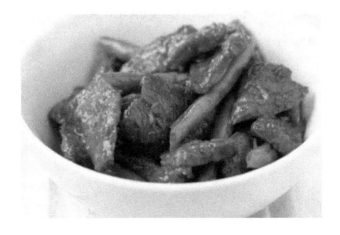

Green Curry Beef

Serves 6 pax

Ingredients

- 1/4 cup fish sauce
- 1 cup basil
- 1/4 cup Green Curry Paste
- 1/4 cup brown sugar pound, cut into 1/4-inch slices
- 6 serrano chilies, stemmed, seeded, and cut in half along the length
- 1 pound sirloin, cut into fine strips
- 2 cans coconut milk, thick cream separated from the milk

Procedure

1. Put the thick cream from the coconut milk and the curry paste in a big soup pot and stir until blended.

2. Put on moderate to high heat and bring to its boiling point. Decrease the heat and simmer for two to three minutes.

3. Put in the beef and the coconut milk, stirring to blend. Return the mixture to a simmer.

4. Put in the sugar and the fish sauce, stirring until the sugar dissolves, approximately 2 minutes.

5. Put in the eggplant and simmer for one to two minutes. Put in the serrano chilies and cook one minute more.

6. Turn off the heat and mix in the basil.

Thai Beef and Broccoli

Serves 4 pax

Ingredients

- 1 medium shallot, chopped
- 1 pound lean beef, cut into bite-sized pieces
- 1/2 of a 7 ounces package of rice sticks
- 1 cup broccoli pieces
- 1 tablespoon preserved soybeans
- 1 teaspoon chili powder
- 3 cups water
- 2 tablespoons vegetable oil
- 1 teaspoon Hot sauce
- 4 lime wedges
- 2 tablespoons brown sugar
- 2 tablespoons fish sauce
- 3 tablespoons sweet soy sauce

Procedure

1. Heat the vegetable oil in a wok on moderate to high heat. Put in the shallot and stir-fry until it starts to become tender.
2. Put in the chili powder and continue to stir-fry until well blended.
3. Put in the brown sugar, fish sauce, soy sauce, and soybeans; stir-fry for half a minute.
4. Put in the beef and continue to stir-fry until the beef is almost done, roughly two minutes.
5. Mix in the water and bring it to its boiling point. Put in the rice sticks, stirring until they start to cook.
6. Lower the heat to moderate, cover, and allow to cook for half a minute. Stir and decrease the heat to moderate-low, cover, and allow to cook for about three minutes.
7. Put in the broccoli pieces, cover, and cook for a minute. Take away the wok from the heat and tweak seasoning to taste.
8. Serve with wedges of lime and hot sauce passed separately at the table.

Grilled Gingered Beef

Serves 6 pax

Ingredients

- 1 (2-inch) piece of ginger, minced
- 1 (3-inch) piece ginger, cut in half
- 1 cinnamon stick
- 1 onion, cut in half
- 1 pound green vegetables
- 1 small package of rice noodles
- 2 dried red chili peppers
- 2 stalks lemongrass
- 2 tablespoons soy sauce
- 2 cloves garlic
- 6 (6-ounce) strip steaks
- 6 scallions, minced
- 8 cups low-salt beef broth
- Salt and pepper to taste

Procedure

1. Put the beef broth, lemongrass, and garlic in a big pot; bring to its boiling point.
2. Meanwhile, put the ginger and onion halves, cut-side down, in a dry frying pan using high heat and cook until black. Put in the onion and ginger to the broth mixture.
3. Put the cinnamon and dried chili peppers in the dry frying pan and toast on moderate heat for a minute; put into the broth mixture.
4. Lower the heat and simmer the broth for a couple of hours. Cool, strain, and place in your fridge overnight.
5. Before you are ready to eat, remove the broth from the fridge and skim off any fat that may have collected.
6. Bring the broth to a simmer and put in the minced ginger.Soak the rice noodles in hot water for ten to twenty minutes or until soft; drain.

7. Blanch the vegetables for approximately one minute. Using a slotted spoon, remove them from the boiling water and shock them in cold water.

8. Season the broth to taste with the soy sauce. Season the steaks with salt and pepper and grill or broil to your preference.

9. To serve, slice the steaks into fine strips (cutting across the grain) and put them in 6 big bowls.

10. Put in a portion of noodles and vegetables to the bowls and ladle the broth over the top.

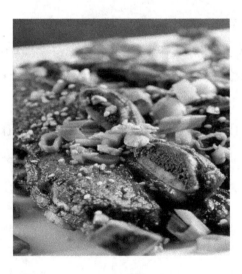

Beef on Rice Noodles

Serves 4 pax

Ingredients

- 1 pound greens (such as spinach or bok choy), cleaned and slice into 1/2-inch strips
- 2 eggs, beaten
- 2 tablespoons dark brown sugar
- 1/4 cup soy sauce
- 5 tablespoons vegetable oil, divided
- 2 crushed dried red pepper flakes to taste
- Freshly ground black pepper
- 1/2 pound dried rice noodles
- 3/4 pound sirloin, trimmed of all fat, washed and patted dry
- 2 tablespoons fish sauce
- 2 tablespoons minced garlic
- Rice vinegar to taste

Procedure

1. Cut the meat into two-inch-long, 1/2–inch-wide strips. Cover the noodles with warm water for five minutes, then drain.

2. In a small container, mix the soy sauce, fish sauce, brown sugar, and black pepper; set aside.

3. Heat a wok or heavy frying pan using high heat. Put in roughly 2 tablespoons of the vegetable oil.

4. Once the oil is hot, but not smoking, put in the garlic. After stirring for 5 seconds, put in the greens and stir-fry for roughly two minutes; set aside.

5. Put in 2 more tablespoons of oil to the wok. Put in the beef and stir-fry until browned on all sides, approximately 2 minutes; set aside.

6. Heat 1 tablespoon of oil in the wok and put in the noodles. Toss until warmed through, roughly two minutes; set aside.

7. Heat the oil remaining in the wok. Put in the eggs and cook, without stirring until they are set, approximately half a minute.

8. Break up the eggs slightly and mix in the reserved noodles, beef, and greens, and the red pepper flakes.

9. Mix the reserved soy mixture, then put in it to the wok. Toss to coat and heat through.

10. Serve instantly with rice vinegar to drizzle over the top.

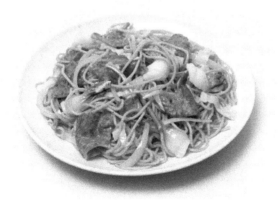

Stir-Fried Minted Beef

Serves 4 pax

Ingredients

- 3 tablespoons fish sauce
- 7 serrano chilies, seeded and crudely chopped
- 1/4 cup chopped garlic
- 1/4 cup chopped yellow or white onion
- 1/2 cup water
- 1/4 cup vegetable oil
- 1/2 cup chopped mint leaves
- 1 pound flank steak, cut across the grain into fine strips
- 1 tablespoon sugar

Procedure

1. Using a mortar and pestle or a food processor, grind together the chilies, garlic, and onion.

2. Heat the oil on moderate to high heat in a wok or big frying pan. Put in the ground chili mixture to the oil and stir-fry for one to two minutes.

3. Put in the beef and stir-fry until it just starts to brown.

4. Put in the rest of the ingredients, adjusting the amount of water depending on how thick you desire the sauce.

5. Serve with sufficient Jasmine rice.

Grilled Beef Tenderloin Steak

Serves 2 pax

Ingredients

- 1/4 teaspoon dried basil
- 1/4 teaspoon dried thyme leaves
- 1 tablespoon Dijon mustard
- 1/2 teaspoons horseradish
- 1/4 teaspoon black pepper
- 2 (8 ounces) beef tenderloin steaks
- 1/4 teaspoon dried tarragon leaves
- Salt to taste

Procedure

1. Stir mustard, horseradish, basil, thyme, tarragon, and pepper to make a paste.
2. Spread paste over top and sides of steaks and wrap each steak in plastic wrap. Marinate steaks in refrigerator overnight.
3. Preheat oven to 400°F. Lightly coat a small, glass baking dish with cooking spray.
4. Unwrap marinated steaks. Season with salt and place in baking dish.
5. Roast steaks to preference (30 minutes for medium-rare, 1 hour for well done).
6. Let rest 5 minutes and serve.

Spicy Beef Stir-Fry

Serves 4 pax

Ingredients

- 2 Tbsp Canola oil
- 2 Tbsp Cilantro, chopped
- 3 Garlic cloves, minced)
- 1 Tbsp Ginger, freshly minced
- 2 Green onions, sliced thinly
- 1 Jalapeno, seeded and sliced thinly
- 1 cup Light coconut milk
- 2 Tbsp Lime juice
- half tsp Lime zest
- Salt and pepper
- 1 lb Sirloin steak, cut into thin strips
- 4 cups Spinach
- 1 Tbsp Sriracha sauce
- 1 Sweet red pepper, cut into thin strips

Procedure

1. Toss the beef, two cloves of garlic, ginger, pepper, and salt in a large container.
2. Allow their flavors to blend for 15 minutes. Separately, whip the coconut milk, chili sauce, lime zest, juice, and salt until well incorporated.
3. Heat a big, oiled pan on medium-high heat. Place your beef inside and fry until cook through. Pull it out of the pan.
4. Fry up the red pepper, jalapeno, red onion, and the last garlic clove with the remaining oil. Cook until the vegetables are crisp-tender.
5. Pour in the coconut milk mixture. Once heated through, toss in the spinach, and reintroduce the beef.
6. Cook until the spinach wilts. When serving, garnish with green onion and cilantro.

Spanish Meatballs in Saffron Soup

Serves 7 pax

Ingredients

For the Meatballs

- 1/2 teaspoon salt
- 1/2 cup Manchego cheese, grated
- 1/3 cup whole milk
- 1/2 teaspoon pepper
- 1 shallot, minced
- 2 tablespoons minced fresh parsley
- 8 ounces 80% lean ground beef
- 8 ounces ground pork
- 7 slices hearty white sandwich bread, torn into quarters
- 2 tablespoons extra-virgin olive oil

For the Soup

- 1 onion, chopped fine
- 1 red bell pepper, stemmed, seeded, and cut into 3/4-inch pieces
- 1/8 teaspoon red pepper flakes
- 2 tablespoons minced fresh parsley
- 8 cups chicken broth
- 1/4 teaspoon saffron threads, crumbled
- 1 cup dry white wine
- 1 tablespoon extra-virgin olive oil
- 1 teaspoon paprika
- 2 garlic cloves, minced
- Salt and pepper

Procedure

For the Meatballs

1. Using fork, mash bread and milk together till it turns into a paste in a big container.
2. Mix in ground pork, Manchego, parsley, shallot, oil, salt, and pepper until combined.

99

3. Put in ground beef and knead with your hands until combined. Pinch off and roll 2-teaspoon-size pieces of mixture into balls and lay out on rimmed baking sheet (you should have 30 to 35 meatballs).

4. Cover using plastic wrap put inside your fridge until firm, minimum 30 minutes.

For the Soup

1. Heat oil in large Dutch oven on moderate to high heat until it starts to shimmer. Put in onion and bell pepper and cook till they become tender and lightly browned, eight to ten minutes.

2. Mix in garlic, paprika, saffron, and pepper flakes and cook until aromatic.

3. Mix in wine, scraping up any browned bits, and cook until almost completely evaporated.

4. Mix in broth and bring to simmer. Gently put in meatballs and simmer until cooked through, 10 to 12 minutes.

5. Remove from the heat, mix in picada and parsley and sprinkle with salt and pepper to taste.

6. Serve.

Thank you, *dear meat lover.*

I am glad you accepted my teachings.

These meals have been personally codified in my worldwide trips.

I wanted to share them with you, to let people know more about meat and how to treat it properly.

Now you had come to know about Beef in all of its shapes, let me give you one more tip.

This manual takes part of an unmissable cookbooks collection.

These meat-based recipes, mixed to all the tastes I met around the world, will give you a complete idea of the possibilities this world offers to us.

You have now the opportunity to add hundreds new elements to your cooking skills knowledge.

Check out the other books!

Dorian Gravy

CPSIA information can be obtained
at www.ICGtesting.com
Printed in the USA
BVHW041123200521
607796BV00014B/2709

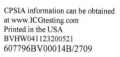